Gut Reset for Women

A Holistic Guide to Heal Your Stomach and Balance Hormones After 50

Omolola Habib

Gut Reset for Women: A Holistic Guide to Heal Your Stomach and Balance Hormones After 50

Copyright © 2024 by **Omolola Habib**

All rights reserved. No part of this publication may be reproduced, distributed, or transmitted in any form or by any means, including photocopying, recording, or other electronic or mechanical methods, without the prior written permission of the publisher, except in the case of brief quotations embodied in critical reviews and certain other noncommercial uses permitted by copyright law.

Table of Content

INTRODUCTION 5

The vital role of your gut — 5

Hormones and digestion, hand in hand — 6

Resetting your gut after 50 — 7

CHAPTER 1: UNDERSTANDING YOUR GUT — 8

Trillions of tiny tenants — 8

What is the gut microbiome and why it's crucial for health — 9

How the gut interacts with the brain, immune system, and hormones — 10

Changes to the gut as we age, especially after 50 — 12

Signs you may have an unhealthy gut — 13

Conclusion — 15

CHAPTER 2: LINK BETWEEN GUT HEALTH AND HORMONES — 17

How estrogen, progesterone, and cortisol impact the gut — 18

Effects of menopause on the microbiome and digestive health — 19

Gut inflammation and leaky gut syndrome — 21

Tips to support healthy hormone balance through the gut — 22

Conclusion — 23

CHAPTER 3: REPAIRING YOUR GUT AFTER 50 — 25

Addressing age-related changes like increased inflammation and decreased diversity — 26

Foods that harm vs. foods that heal your gut after 50   27

Lifestyle factors like sleep, stress, exercise   29

Supplements that support gut health during menopause   30

Conclusion   31

CHAPTER 4: THE GUT HEALTH DIET   33

Overview of Eating for Optimal Gut Health   33

Avoiding Common Triggers like Gluten, Dairy, Sugar   38

Focusing on Anti-Inflammatory Foods, Fiber, Fermented Foods   42

Sample Meal Plan and Recipes   46

Conclusion   56

CHAPTER 5: LIFESTYLE CHANGES FOR BETTER GUT HEALTH   61

Managing stress and cortisol levels   61

Getting regular exercise and restorative sleep   63

Supporting gut microbes through meditation, nature   64

Probiotics and prebiotics   65

CONCLUSION   67

Key takeaways   67

Putting it all together for an optimal gut reset   68

Looking ahead to healthier aging   69

ABOUT THE AUTHOR   71

Introduction

As we age, our gut health tends to decline - but women need to take care of theirs after 50. The truth is, that so much of our overall well-being depends on the state of our digestive system. Yet it's often overlooked or underappreciated.

In this book, I hope to change that by bringing focus to this crucial aspect of health and wellness. You'll learn exactly how your gut influences more than just digestion - it's truly intertwined with your entire being and sense of balance. With some simple lifestyle shifts, you have the power to reverse certain changes, heal imbalances, and feel your very best well into your later years.

The vital role of your gut

Modern research has shown us that the gut is far more than just a pathway for food. At its core lies a complex ecosystem containing trillions of microscopic organisms known as your gut microbiome. This diverse community plays a leading role in everything from immune function to brain health to metabolism.

Scientists now understand that 90% of serotonin - one of the main hormones linked to mood - is synthesized in the gastrointestinal tract. Your gut also communicates bidirectionally with your brain via the gut-brain axis, allowing intestinal bacteria to influence neurological processes. No wonder optimal digestive wellness is so strongly tied to mental wellbeing.

The gut microbiome is shaped by much more than diet alone; factors like stress levels, age, and genetics all leave their mark. This means as we age and go through life's ups and downs, microbiome composition naturally transforms. And for women, the hormonal rollercoaster of menopause brings its own set of changes to further impact gut ecology.

Lack of diversity in gut bacteria has been associated with numerous health issues from autoimmune diseases to cancer risk. Digestive disturbances like gas, bloating, constipation, or diarrhea can also seriously impact the quality of life - and tend to flare up more frequently post-50. By supporting a rich, balanced gut microcosm, you set the foundation for vitality on multiple levels.

Hormones and digestion, hand in hand

Women's hormones are deeply intertwined with our digestion in ways that are only now coming into focus. Estrogen, progesterone, and other "sex hormones" play a significant role in maintaining gastrointestinal function and barrier integrity. They influence motility, secretion, inflammation levels, and much more.

As hormone production shifts dramatically with perimenopause and menopause, these effects ripple throughout the entire digestive system. Common issues like slower metabolism, altered bowel habits, and digestive sensitivity often emerge or intensify as a result. Additionally, an imbalance in the gut microbiome may feed back to disrupt hormonal balance even further in the form of dysbiosis or "bad" bacterial overgrowth.

It's clear how this cycle of dysregulation can perpetuate health issues for postmenopausal women. The good news is that empowering your gut has proven benefits of stabilizing mood, reducing disease risk and even counteracting some unpleasant menopausal symptoms. By taking a holistic approach with diet, lifestyle interventions, and targeted supplements when needed, you can support your gut-hormone health in tandem as you age.

Resetting your gut after 50

I am so excited to share this book with you as your guide to gut resetting. Throughout the next chapters, you'll gain a deeper understanding of how your digestive ecosystem works and the many ways you can optimize it through the years of menopause and beyond.

We'll explore the specific gut changes that often come with aging, like shifting microbiota and heightened levels of oxidative stress and inflammation. You'll learn to identify potential problem areas through gut-health symptom awareness. Then we'll unlock practical strategies for replenishing your microbiome diversity and rebuilding gut integrity.

I hope that by making small, sustainable changes to your diet, supplements, and daily routines, you can feel empowered guardianship over your health as the year progresses. With an easy-to-follow reset plan tailored just for you, this book will equip you to navigate age-related transformation from the inside out - starting with your beautiful, versatile gut.

I'm thrilled to share this knowledge and guide you on your path to whole-body wellness. Let's get started!

Chapter 1: Understanding Your Gut

Now that we've gotten an overview of how crucial gut health is, it's time to take a deeper look into what your gut is. In this chapter, we'll explore the complex intestinal ecosystem known as your microbiome and digestion down to the cellular level. My goal is to give you an appreciation for just how intricate and vital this often-overlooked organ system truly is.

With knowledge comes empowerment, so consider this your first step to gaining mastery over your gut wellness. You'll find that understanding how everything fits together from bacteria to bile will also help you recognize potential trouble spots as you continue your reset journey. So let's start at the very beginning - it's time to meet your mighty microbiome!

Trillions of tiny tenants

If you could peer inside your gut, you'd find it buzzing with microorganisms - bacteria, viruses, yeasts, and more all calling your intestines home. The bacterial portion alone numbers around 100 trillion, collectively comprising a weight of around 3 pounds! This mass of microscopic life dwelling within you is appropriately referred to as your gut microbiome.

You may be surprised to learn that genetically, your microbiome contains over 100 times as many genes as your actual human DNA. Inhabiting your entire gastrointestinal tract from mouth to anus, these commensal organisms perform functions you quite literally could not survive without. From nutrient synthesis to digestion to immunity, your intimate gut tenets play an outsized role in your day-to-day health and well-being.

It turns out we have co-evolved with our microbiome for millions of years in a symbiotic relationship of mutual benefit. Their metabolic activity allows us to harvest calories and nutrients from foods in ways our human genomes lack the capacity for alone. Meanwhile, our digestive tract offers them shelter, sustenance, and a stable environment to thrive. Win-win!

Your gut bacterial communities also act as a living barrier against pathogens, train your immune defenses from a young age, and converse with your brain using neurotransmitters to influence everything from mood to appetite. As you can see, your microbial tenants are far from passive passengers - they actively participate in your physiological processes each moment of every day.

What is the gut microbiome and why it's crucial for health

Now that we have an idea of just how many tiny tenants call our digestive tracts home, it's important to define what exactly is meant by the term "gut microbiome". In essence, it refers to the entire collective genome composed of all the microorganisms inhabiting our intestines.

While this includes various types of microbes, the dominant residents by far are bacteria - with over 500 different species identified so far. Each person's profile differs, but a healthy microbiome usually contains several dominant types such as Bifidobacteria and Lactobacillus that aid digestion and support our immune defenses.

The diversity and balance of these microbes are incredibly impactful. Their combined metabolic activity allows us to extract vitamins, minerals, antioxidants, and short-chain fatty acids from our foods that benefit us in numerous ways:

- Energy harvest - Bacteria ferment fibers into nutrients like butyrate, which provides around 10% of an adult's daily calorie needs.

- Immunity - They educate our immune cells from a young age and fight to maintain gut barrier integrity. A healthy balance deters the overgrowth of pathogenic invaders.

- Neurology - As mentioned, neurotransmitter signaling between microbes and our enteric nervous system can influence mood, appetite, and pain sensitivity.

- Inflammation - Certain bacteria secrete anti-inflammatory compounds while others induce regulatory immune cells to prevent issues like IBS, colitis, or inflammatory bowel disease if kept in check.

As you can see, our gut flora plays roles as diverse as our energy levels, defense mechanisms, mental well-being, and physical health. Nurturing a richness and stability of microbiota is truly vital self-care with far-reaching impacts throughout the entire body.

How the gut interacts with the brain, immune system, and hormones

At this point, we understand the gut microbiome is vital to overall wellness - but its role extends far beyond just digestion. Let's dig deeper into how your intestinal tenants truly interface with every major bodily system from brain to immunity to endocrine function.

The gut-brain connection

Two-way communication exists between your gut and brain via the vagus nerve, hormones, and active neurotransmitters. Microbes can signal hunger, cravings, moods, and more up to the brain. Meanwhile, stress and emotions directed down from the brain influence gut physiology and microbial populations. This bidirectional "gut-brain axis" plays a major role in conditions like anxiety, depression, Alzheimer's, and more.

Immune system liaison

Around 70% of your immune cells reside in the gastrointestinal tract. Gut bacteria guide immune cell development and regulate inflammation responses. They produce compounds that train immune cells to tolerate commensal microbes while attacking invaders. This immune education and balanced pro/anti-inflammatory activity are central to preventing autoimmune disorders, food sensitivity, and infection risk.

Hormonal interplay

The gut manufactures serotonin as mentioned, but also influences testosterone and estrogen levels. Probiotic metabolites engage with hormone receptors throughout our bodies. Meanwhile, reproductive and stress hormones like progesterone, cortisol, and DHEA shape the microbial ecosystem. Their interplay grows more complex during stages like menopause transitioning. Supporting a balanced microbiota may help moderate common hormonal imbalance symptoms.

It's mind-blowing to grasp your digestive tract is truly a full-fledged organ system interacting intimately with every other physiological process in your body. With a foundational understanding of these complex relationships, you can appreciate how empowering gut health choices encompasses your whole self at the deepest levels.

Changes to the gut as we age, especially after 50

While a healthy gut microbiome tends to remain relatively stable through adulthood, aging does bring about some natural shifts that can compromise its balance over time if left unaddressed. For women in particular, transitions in the later decades present additional microbial challenges.

As early as our 40s, microbial diversity may gradually narrow as certain species become less prevalent with age. Concurrently, facultative anaerobes like Enterococcus which are typically in low amounts may expand their population somewhat. Both trends correlate with mild inflammation and digestive changes.

However, research indicates gut changes can accelerate more noticeably in women's 50s and beyond. For instance:

- Declining estrogen can thin intestinal walls, raising permeability or "leaky gut" risk which allows undigested particles into the bloodstream, fueling systemic inflammation.

- Slower motility due to aging and menopause often leads to constipation if dietary fiber intake isn't increased to compensate.

- Lower antioxidant defenses invite more oxidative stress damage to gut cells and DNA of resident microbes over the decades.

- Stress hormones rise as adrenal function shifts, which can favor the growth of opportunistic bacteria better able to withstand cortisol surges that healthier strains may struggle with.

While these shifts are normal to a degree as the years progress, the good news is dietary and lifestyle tweaks have proven very effective at supporting a healthier microbial profile well into advanced age. Making gut-nurturing choices now can help counteract inevitable changes.

Signs you may have an unhealthy gut

Now that we've explored the crucial role and typical aging dynamics of the gastrointestinal system, let's highlight some potential red flags that could indicate your gut isn't as balanced as it could be. Being aware of these common symptoms will help you determine if you may benefit from implementing a reset plan.

Digestive issues are notoriously tricky to pin down, so don't panic if you relate to just one or two - everybody is unique. But noticing a cluster of these signs, especially if new or intensifying as the years pass, is reason enough to take proactive steps to investigate further and nourish your gut ecology:

- Bloating, gas, or abdominal discomfort after meals that impair daily activities. This could point to food sensitivities, low stomach acid, or dysbiosis.

- Changes in bowel habits like diarrhea or constipation alternating, or stools that are loose, hard, pale, greasy, or contain undigested food particles may signify malabsorption problems or imbalances throughout the gut.

- Indigestion, acid reflux, or nausea that brings distress and interferes with sleep quality. This can stem from low stomach acid, hiatal hernia, or inflammation.

- Chronic fatigue that doesn't improve with rest. An exhausted microbiome may struggle to produce vitamins and isn't as effective at breaking down foods for energy retrieval.

- Recurrent infections, sinus issues, or urinary tract problems as an imbalanced microbiota is less apt to prevent pathogen overgrowth and maintain sterile environments where needed.

- Mood changes like anxiety, depression, brain fog, or difficulty concentrating. Bidirectional communication issues on the gut-brain axis are one potential explanation.

- Skin conditions such as acne, eczema, or psoriasis as gut dysbiosis allow excessive inflammation and nutrient malabsorption systemically.

- Unexplained weight fluctuations in either direction. Your metabolism and nutrient yields from foods depend on optimized digestion.

Ruling out other health factors, and addressing underlying causes of multiple signs through lifestyle and diet can work wonders for rediscovering energetic, balanced wellness from within.

Conclusion

I hope this examination into the marvelous complexity of your gastrointestinal system has left you with an even deeper appreciation for the gut-body connection. From the trillions of microscopic allies inhabiting your intestines to their multidirectional interfaces throughout your physiology - it's astounding to reflect on the integral role digestion plays in overall wellness.

Seeing as 90% of serotonin production and up to 70% of your immune system is gut-based, among many other vital functions, it's no exaggeration to say that empowering your digestive health amounts to empowering your entire self down to the cellular level. With aging especially, proactive efforts to support gut resilience will tangibly impact your energy, immunity, and disease risk for years to come.

Some key takeaways to contemplate moving forward:

- Your gut microbiome is diverse, interactive, and co-evolved for health alongside changing microbiota across a lifetime.

- Microbial imbalance can manifest mentally or physically in every major system from the brain to the skin through mechanisms like inflammation, nutrient status, and microbial communication.

- While shifts occur naturally with aging, especially during menopause, diet, and lifestyle choices make an impact in countering atrophy to resilience.

- Symptom awareness is empowering for recognizing potential dysbiosis in its earlier stages before a cascade of issues takes hold.

Our journey has only just begun! In upcoming chapters, we'll explore targeting common post-menopausal gut disruptions like leaky gut, hormone fluctuations, and microbial shift. You'll gain practical guidance toward individualized healing through targeted nutrition, supplements, and daily habits.

I hope you now feel greater empowerment to proactively support this often overlooked yet profoundly vital organ system. Let's continue unlocking wisdom and starting your customized gut reset approach!

Chapter 2: Link Between Gut Health and Hormones

In our first chapter, we explored the intricate workings of your gut and microbiome. Now that we understand this system's profound influence throughout the body, it's time to zoom in on its specific connections to another key aspect of female health - hormones.

As dynamic as the gut is complex, so too are our endocrine processes, especially during stages like perimenopause and menopause. These years bring about immense transformation from our teens through natural bodily changes. Within this adaptive time, supporting gut function takes on increasing significance for our overall well-being.

Let's deepen our knowledge of exactly how gut microbiota and hormones engage in constant dialogue. An optimally balanced microbiome plays a leading role in moderating our hormone levels, activity, and reception across target tissues. Meanwhile, hormones like estrogen shape our intestinal flora.

When this intricate relationship falters, so too can numerous aspects of our health like mood, metabolism, and disease risk. However, empowering our gut ecosystem through small daily adjustments proves remarkably effective for counteracting imbalances brought by the hormonal transition.

In this chapter, I hope that gaining insights into the two-way gut-hormone street will inspire you to nurture this connection however suits your unique needs. An integrated approach addressing both domains nourishes wellness at a deep, multi-system level through life's ever-changing seasons.

So without further ado, let's embark on exploring the intricate interplay between your gut microbiome and the hormones that guide your extraordinary female journey!

How estrogen, progesterone, and cortisol impact the gut

Our major "sex hormones" estrogen and progesterone are perhaps most recognized for their regulation of the menstrual cycle and role in reproductive processes. However, their influence also profoundly impacts the bowel thanks to abundant receptors within the gut wall and enteric nervous system.

Estrogen in particular helps maintain gut function in several key ways:

- It supports intestinal barrier integrity by up-regulating tight junction proteins that seal spaces between intestinal cells. This protects against dietary antigens and endotoxins that can otherwise leak into circulation.

- Peristalsis and motility are modulated, aiding proper digestion transit time and bowel elimination. Changes here as estrogen levels drop may cause constipation for some.

- Inflammation is suppressed through interactions that down-regulate pro-inflammatory cytokines and oxidative damage throughout the digestive tract.

Meanwhile, progesterone encourages the absorption of important minerals like calcium and magnesium through intestinal transport mechanisms and fluid secretions aiding nutrient uptake. It also fosters a balanced microbiota partly through antioxidant effects.

As for cortisol, this stress hormone rises during aging partly due to shifting adrenal function. While temporary surges protectively mobilize energy during fight or flight, chronic high cortisol corrodes gut health in a few key ways:

- It thins intestinal walls, compromising barrier integrity through the breakdown of tight junction proteins as seen with prolonged stress.

- Immune function is modulated towards a pro-inflammatory profile through cortisol receptor interactions on immune cells in the Gut-Associated Lymphoid Tissue (GALT).

- Microbial dysbiosis occurs with repeated cortisol spikes favoring opportunistic "bad" bacteria over symbiotic strains more cortisol-sensitive.

Optimizing sex hormone and cortisol balance through lifestyle self-care and dietary support thus proves vital for protecting gastrointestinal function, especially as levels shift with menopause. A balanced gut flora also modulates these hormones in turn, as we will discuss.

Effects of menopause on the microbiome and digestive health

While shifts occur naturally as we age, the hormonal upheaval accompanying menopause transition presents additional challenges for maintaining gut equilibrium. Estrogen's decline especially impacts intestinal functions in ways correlating with common menopausal digestive symptoms.

Microbial dysbiosis has been documented in menopause, with studies finding lower counts of "good" Bifidobacterium and Lactobacillus that aid digestion. Concurrently, opportunistic bacteria like Clostridium perfringens are more abundant - which promotes inflammatory profiles.

Specific factors contributing to microbiome changes include:

- Estrogen depletion permits greater gut wall permeability due to the breakdown of tight junction proteins. This exposes bacteria to immune cells in the gut lining, fueling dysregulated inflammation.

- Changes in digestion like slower transit time and irregular bowel habits as peristalsis weaken without estrogen's moderating effects. This enables bacteria to overgrow in the bowel.

- Drops in antioxidants that bacteria depend on for viability, as menopause diminishes physiological defenses against oxidative stress and cellular damage.

- Increase in pathogenic bacteria as probiotic strains succumb to a higher redox environment and weaker epithelial barrier through the large intestine.

Resulting microbial imbalances translate to digestive issues plaguing many women, such as bloating, gas, constipation, diarrhea, leaky gut, and IBS. Belly discomfort is one of menopause's most prevalent reported symptoms, with prevalence doubling during peri-menopause.

Other common problems like acid reflux, ulcerative colitis, and bowel inflammation also seem more common in post-menopausal women following shifts in hormone levels, microbial metabolites, and gut immunity. Rebalancing the inner ecosystem helps counter these evolving difficulties.

Gut inflammation and leaky gut syndrome

As discussed, hormonal shifts impact the gastrointestinal lining through factors like weakened tight junctions and an imbalanced microbiota inclined towards pro-inflammatory patterns. These changes promote gut inflammation and contribute to "leaky gut syndrome" - a condition with important implications for health.

When intestinal permeability increases, usually as a result of chronic inflammation, it allows undigested food particles, toxins, and microbes to pass from inside the gut into surrounding tissues and bloodstream where they don't belong. This triggers an immune reaction systemically.

Some additional factors driving gut inflammation and increased permeability during menopause include:

- Loss of estrogen's anti-inflammatory actions on intestinal cells
- Changes in microbial metabolites like bacterially-produced LPS endotoxins as bacterial populations alter
- Higher systemic inflammation influenced by adipose tissue as weight distributes after menopause
- Stress hormone elevation, especially long-term, damages the gut epithelium

Consequences of this "leaky gut" effect include food sensitivities developing, autoimmune tendencies, fatigue, brain fog, skin issues, and weight fluctuations as the body redirects blood flow and resources to cope with the immune response. It has been linked to digestive disorders, heart disease, diabetes, and even mental health conditions.

Healing and sealing the gut lining through targeted nutrients, reducing inflammatory foods/lifestyle triggers, and repopulating with symbiotic bacteria are pivotal for counteracting these age-related changes. An anti-inflammatory microbiota correlates closely with hormone balance through multiple avenues.

Tips to support healthy hormone balance through the gut

By now we can appreciate the depth of interplay between our intestinal ecosystem and hormone functions - especially as changes occur during life stages like perimenopause. The good news is that simple dietary tweaks and lifestyle habits have great potential to positively influence this relationship.

Nourishing a robust, balanced gut flora promotes hormone balance through a few key mechanisms:

- Certain probiotics secrete bioactive compounds like equol and enterolignans that engage with estrogen receptors similarly to plant estrogens. This modulates cellular response and helps regulate normal hormonal activity.

- Bacterial metabolites interact with the HPA axis and hypothalamus to help control stress responses. Lower cortisol levels aid other endocrine functions.

- Short-chain fatty acids like butyrate produced by fiber fermentation support a healthy gut lining, reducing systemic inflammation linked to imbalances.

- Optimizing the gut-brain axis through probiotics, and prebiotics, and managing stress helps restore proper communication between the neurological and endocrine systems.

Some effective strategies that support both the microbiome and hormone balance include:

- Consuming fermented foods daily for probiotic/prebiotic intake
- Including fiber-rich cruciferous vegetables and Limiting sugar
- Staying hydrated to aid digestion and natural bodily functions
- Managing stress with activities like gentle walking, meditation, or journaling
- Getting quality sleep and mobility through daily activity
- Supplementing with targeted probiotics, prebiotics, and nutrients to fill any dietary gaps

Making small changes now through this integrated approach can tangibly improve your well-being. By empowering communication along the gut-hormone highway, you nourish balance from within during life's transitions.

Conclusion

If this chapter underscored anything, it's the profound depth and mutual influence between our gastrointestinal and hormonal domains. Through dynamic interactions at the gut microbiome, intestinal, and whole body levels, these two physiological networks engage in constant cross-talk shaping our wellness from within.

This two-way street takes on heightened significance during midlife hormonal transitions. But knowledge is empowering, and making simple self-care adjustments to common challenges can go far in counteracting imbalance. By approaching gut and hormone support together through dietary optimization and stress management, exponential benefits multiply.

Before moving forward, here are a few key takeaways:

- Estrogen, progesterone, and cortisol profoundly impact the gut, and gut flora modulate these hormones in turn.

- Menopause translates to digestion difficulty partly due to declining intestinal health support from estrogen and microbiome shifts.

- Leaky gut and systemic inflammation intensify without measures to reduce triggers and seal the barrier.

- Certain probiotic forms engage with hormone receptors, while others control stress pathways.

- Meal choices, hydration, activity, sleep, and relaxing techniques reinforce this relationship.

With a mindset of nurturing communication along the entire gut-hormone pathway, the coming insights in Chapter 3 will guide individualizing your approach through purposeful nutrition and targeted supplements. Your self-care represents an investment in radiant well-being for years ahead. Let's continue our journey towards balance!

Chapter 3: Repairing Your Gut After 50

By now we understand the gut microbiome is dynamic yet subtly altered through natural aging and hormonal shifts. While some change is inevitable, the encouraging message is that dietary interventions pack remarkable healing power to restore balance from within during menopause.

In this chapter, we delve into how certain lifestyle and nutrition choices positively reinforce your inner ecosystem against typical difficulties emerging post-50 like weakened gut lining integrity and microbial imbalance. You'll gain insights for mitigating inflammation, optimizing digestion function, and rewilding your microbiota diversity through purposeful daily self-care.

Rather than fearing hormonal transitions, view them as an opportunity to empower gut resilience and prevent long-term issues down the line. Small adjustments compounded over time yield tremendous effects through a process of patient restoration. Think of it as gardening for the trillions of microbes supporting total well-being behind the scenes.

By learning to recognize lifestyle influences within and outside your control, you can adjust environments and habits customized to your changing needs. An anti-aging gut begins with informed choices guiding renewed gut-hormone communication each day.

It's now time to explore tailored strategies for healing, fueling, and friend-making within your gut landscape! Let's discover pathways welcoming vibrant wellness from the inside out.

Addressing age-related changes like increased inflammation and decreased diversity

Two physiological shifts that are typical with aging yet exacerbated by menopause are increased gut and systemic inflammation, as well as declining microbial diversity within the intestines. Targeting these shifts through diet is foundational for gut and overall health optimization at this stage.

Choosing whole, high-fiber, antioxidant-rich foods starves inflammation naturally:

- Fermentable fibers fuel beneficial bacteria to produce short-chain fatty acids like butyrate, which reduce gut wall inflammation and nourish colon cells. Good sources include legumes, oats, and vegetables.

- Phytonutrients and plant compounds in berries, herbs, spices, dark leafy greens, tomatoes, and broccoli family vegetables quench oxidative damage to cells and DNA linked to the aging process.

- Omega-3 fats from fatty fish, flax, and chia seeds, as well as nuts and seeds, tamp down excess inflammation while supporting a robust epithelial gut lining.

Consuming varied prebiotics lets microbes self-select healthier strains better able to resist environmental stresses. Probiotic foods like yogurt, kefir, kimchi, and kombucha introduce symbiotic friends to reinforce diversity as well:

- Rotating daily probiotic sources touches on a range of microbial strains with differing strengths for balanced gut function.

- Prebiotics act as fertilizer for existing bacterial populations to expand, repopulating your inner ecosystem.

The synergistic combination of fiber, antioxidants, omega-3s, prebiotics, and probiotics through whole foods makes a simple yet strategic mealtime-centered approach for gut resetting. With consistency, inflammation quiets while diversity thrives naturally again.

Foods that harm vs. foods that heal your gut after 50

Just as certain whole foods deliver targeted healing benefits, some all-too-common menu items contribute to dysfunction as we age. Recognizing potentially damaging foods empowers substitution for renewed vitality over time.

Foods to limit:

- Sugars and refined carbs feed "bad" bacteria and yeasts, raising inflammation levels within hours through reactions that increase oxidative stress and leaky gut risk over time.

- Processed vegetable/seed/nut oils subject to oxidation at high temperatures like canola, corn, and soybean oils should be swapped for olive oil or MCT oil in limited amounts.

- Artificial sweeteners alter gut flora balance even in small amounts according to research. Best left avoided.

- Excessive alcohol stresses the liver while disrupting microbial balance, barrier integrity, and hydration across bodily systems as we age.

- Highly salted snacks or cured/smoked meats burden the kidneys and cardiovascular system when consumed frequently long-term.

Foods that heal:

- Fermented foods replenish healthy flora through probiotic-rich options like yogurt, kefir, kimchi, kombucha, sauerkraut and tempeh.

- Prebiotic fibers from cruciferous veggies, berries, onions, garlic, asparagus, bananas, and legumes fertilize existing symbiotic colonies.

- Bone broths, gelatin, and collagen support gut lining integrity through proteins nourishing epithelial cell regeneration.

- Anti-inflammatory spices like turmeric, ginger, garlic, and hot peppers alleviate digestion discomfort.

- Fatty fish, walnuts, and flax/chia seeds nourish the body with omega-3s while easing inflammation throughout.

By rotating these gut-healing superstars and minding potentially irritating foods, your inner ecosystem finds renewed balance over the weeks and months to blossom radiantly.

Lifestyle factors like sleep, stress, exercise

While nutrition forms a cornerstone of gut healing, daily stressors exact their toll requiring addressed habits to reinforce wellness. Here are lifestyle priorities for empowering gut and hormone resilience during menopause:

Manage stress

As cortisol rises with stress, relaxation techniques safeguard inner harmony. Emotional freedom techniques (EFT), meditation, and quality time with loved ones boost mood while reducing stress hormones' corrosive effects.

Prioritize sleep

Aim for 7-9 hours nightly as poor sleep promotes systemic inflammation and microbial imbalances. Develop a bedtime routine without screen time to optimize natural circadian rhythms.

Move your body

Whether through walks, water aerobics, dance, or strength training, daily activity stimulates peristalsis, reduces constipation, and balances hormones through endorphins. Plus, exercise calms stress responses over time.

Hydrate properly

Sip water throughout the day to aid digestion and elimination. When dehydrated, the gut pulls moisture from surrounding tissues disrupting microbe viability and barrier integrity.

Limit tobacco and excess alcohol

Both are potent stressors that alter flora balance and increase intestinal wall permeability when consumed frequently.

Cultivate community

Strong social ties naturally relieve stress while fostering a more positive mindset. Gather family/friends regularly for laughter and support.

Prioritizing these aspects of self-care holistically addresses both physical and emotional well-being for radiance emanating from a sense of inner peace and empowerment. Nourish balance through nourishment of body and spirit alike.

Supplements that support gut health during menopause

For some women, lifestyle and dietary adjustments alone may not prove sufficient to fully support gut barrier integrity, microbial balance, and related health priorities during hormonal shifts. In these cases, targeted supplementation offers valuable backup.

Probiotics

Look for broad-spectrum, refrigerated blends containing 30-50 billion CFUs daily of Lactobacillus and Bifidobacterium strains to reinforce beneficial colonies depleted by age and hormones.

Prebiotics

Fiber supplements like inulin, acacia fiber, and psyllium or prebiotic blends encourage gut flora diversification through foods lacking in modern diets.

L-Glutamine

This amino acid supports epithelial barrier health and reduces whole-body inflammation by strengthening intestinal cell junctions and the metabolism of gut immune cells.

Fish oil

EPA and DHA aid an anti-inflammatory gut lining and systemic function through omega-3 fatty acids vital for cell signaling and metabolism.

Turmeric or ginger

Curcumin and gingerols lend antioxidant support to counter menopause-linked oxidative stress and damage tarnishing cells and DNA over time.

Proteolytic enzymes

Enzymes like bromelain, papain, and fungal proteases aid digestive capacity and bloating by breaking down proteins into easily absorbable forms.

Herbal bitters

Gentian, schizandra, and dandelion extracts optimize stomach acid and liver function for maximal nutrient extraction and detox pathways through phytometabolites.

Including carefully chosen supplements under medical guidance individualizes support beyond lifestyle and diet to proactively counter gut imbalances from within over the long term.

Conclusion

By now it should be abundantly clear that targeted dietary choices, lifestyle habits, and natural supplements when chosen carefully offer profound yet gentle support for overall gut resiliency and function approaching midlife and beyond. Whether fighting inflammation, optimizing elimination, or reestablishing microbial allies - these health-driven adjustments impart real transformation over time.

Seeing the gut as a dynamic inner ecosystem to nurture, rather than an afterthought, proves key for radiating wellness multidimensionally during changing seasons. A focus on gut-directed self-care minimizes new issues surfacing while renewing luminous vitality from within.

As we prepare to wrap up foundational blocks for optimizing this crucible of our total health, here are a few takeaways:

- Dietary tweaks minimize inflammation and maximize microbial diversity natural to aging guts.
- Key gut-supportive foods heal while limiting problematic options to remove irritants.
- Lifestyle priorities like managing stress, sufficient sleep, and activity calm cortisol and gut motility.
- Supplements targeted to fill nutritional gaps provide extra backing as needed.

By learning to recognize your self-care influences both within and beyond your control, you gain daily empowerment over your unique transition. Let the journey of steady gut healing and renewal continue!

Chapter 4: The Gut Health Diet

Now that we've explored foundational concepts for targeted gut repair, it's time to apply our learning through a comprehensive meal plan addressing your specific needs at this phase of life's journey.

While constant change and variety nourish the microbiome, following dietary guidelines customized to your goals provides structure during the transition. This chapter presents a sample comprehensive lifestyle plan for you to adapt uniquely.

Our gut health diet centers nutrition around naturally anti-inflammatory, high-fiber whole foods and mindfully chosen supplements. With sustenance focusing on mind, body, and spirit's empowered alignment, radiance blooms effectively within weeks and months of commitment.

This is by no means a rigid prescription, but rather guidance for you to freely work with. Listen to your body, adjust accordingly, and celebrate progress proudly made through small steady steps. Confidence grows as inner wisdom leads the way to vibrant health sustained long-term.

Within you reside innate resources for well-being during any life phase. Let this chapter serve as a starting point to unlock fuller potential at a deeply nourishing level. Make connections between daily choices and your experience with an attitude of care, compassion, and gratitude. Your journey of self-discovery awaits!

Overview of Eating for Optimal Gut Health

A balanced, anti-inflammatory diet that nurtures your gut microbiota is essential for healing persistent digestive problems and promoting general wellbeing. Adopting a "gut-friendly" eating style, however, entails more than only sticking to a diet plan.

It's all about knowing how various nutrients interact with your intestines' sensitive ecosystem. It involves making deliberate decisions that support microbial diversity and eliminate stressors that support dysbiosis and inflammation.

At its core, an optimal gut diet emphasizes:

1) Removing inflammatory, disruptive foods
2) Increasing intake of prebiotic fibers
3) Replenishing with probiotic foods
4) Providing nutrient density for gut healing

Let's explore each of these aspects in more depth:

Removing Inflammatory Foods

As was covered in the previous section, the intestinal lining and microbiota are harmed by specific food groups that act as irritants, such as gluten, dairy, sugar, processed foods, alcohol, and inflammatory oils. They increase the permeability of the stomach, which lets bacteria and partially digested food particles into the bloodstream.

These foreign substances cause the body to launch an inflammatory autoimmune reaction in an attempt to combat and eliminate the perceived threats. The symptoms of this underlying chronic inflammation eventually show themselves as bloating, pain, exhaustion, skin problems, mood disorders, and more.

Eliminating these inflammatory factors for at least 30 days is the first step in a gut reset, which will help put out the fire. An elimination diet offers a fresh start, allowing inflammatory gut tissues to recover and your microbiota to return to balance.

Increasing Prebiotic Fibers

Prebiotics are dietary fibers that support the "good" probiotic bacteria that are already present in your digestive system. They operate as fertilizer, promoting the growth and reestablishment of dominance of advantageous strains such as Lactobacillus and Bifidobacteria.

Top prebiotic fibers include:

- Inulin and FOS from onions, garlic, asparagus, artichokes
- GOS in beans, soy products, cashews, pistachios
- Pectins in apples, berries, citrus fruits, carrots
- Resistant starches from cooled cooked starches (potatoes, pasta, rice)
- Beta-glucans in oats, mushrooms, seaweed

Your gut microbes eat these indigestible fibers as they pass through the small intestine and into the colon. The bacteria generate short-chain fatty acids like butyrate through this fermentation process, which lowers inflammation and nourishes gut cells.

Increasing your prebiotic consumption also helps you feel fuller after meals, have regular bowel movements, and absorb minerals better.

Replenishing with Probiotic Foods

Probiotic foods offer a fresh source of live, beneficial bacterial strains to help swiftly re-establish a strong, diverse microbiome, while prebiotics work as fuel for bacteria. Among the best sources of probiotics are:

- Fermented dairy: Kefir, yogurt, aged cheeses
- Fermented vegetables: Sauerkraut, kimchi, pickles
- Fermented soy: Tempeh, miso, natto
- Other fermented foods: Kombucha, apple cider vinegar, kvass
- Probiotic supplements with diverse Lactobacillus/Bifidobacterium strains

These living organisms help by:

- Producing vitamins, enzymes, and antioxidants
- Crowding out harmful microbes and pathogens
- Supporting the intestinal barrier and gut immunity
- Enhancing digestion and mineral absorption
- Detoxifying BPAs, heavy metals, and carcinogenic compounds
- Modulating hormones, neurotransmitters, and anti-inflammatory compounds

Start slowly by incorporating small portions of fermented foods daily and rotating between different varieties. This allows your gut to adapt to new bacterial colonies gently.

Over time, increase your intake for maximum probiotic diversity.

Emphasizing Nutrient-Density

Feeding your gut a wide array of colorful, nutrient-dense plant foods and healthy proteins creates the ideal nutritional environment to facilitate healing. Some key nutrients for gut health include:

- Anti-inflammatory fats: Omega-3s, olive oil, avocados, nuts, seeds
- Antioxidants: Berries, leafy greens, broccoli, turmeric
- L-glutamine: Nourishes intestinal cells
- Zinc: Supports gut immunity and cell regeneration
- Vitamins A, C, and E: Enhance gut barrier integrity
- Bone broth: Supplies gut-healing collagen, gelatin, glycine

These micronutrients reinforce tight junctions, promote immunological function and detoxification, reduce inflammation, improve gut motility, and regenerate intestinal tissues.

Achieving a sufficient intake of soluble and insoluble fiber from fruits, vegetables, nuts, and whole grains is equally important. Microbes are fed by soluble fibers, whereas insoluble fibers give regularity by adding mass.

Remember to stay properly hydrated by drinking lots of filtered water, herbal teas, and soothing liquids like bone broth. Maintaining a balanced fluid intake is essential for softer stools and avoidance of constipation.

As you can see, consuming fermented foods and avoiding gluten is only one aspect of a complete gut-healing diet. Instead, it's a deliberate, multifaceted approach to establishing an environment within the body that is rich in nutrients for repair and regeneration, microbiome-friendly, and anti-inflammatory.

Adapt your meals to your individual dietary sensitivities and make these principles your compass. You'll be surprised at how quickly and significantly your gut health improves!

Avoiding Common Triggers like Gluten, Dairy, Sugar

Not all foods work the same way when it comes to repairing the gut and restoring balance to your microbiota. Some commonplace staple foods can worsen gut problems by acting as inflammatory triggers. We'll look at some of the main offenders in this part and explain why it's so important to minimize or stay away from them.

Gluten

Grain varieties such as wheat, barley, rye, and triticale contain the protein gluten. Although not intrinsically harmful, it might cause issues for a lot of people for the reasons listed below:

- **Leaky Gut**: Gluten contains proteins like gliadin that promote intestinal permeability or "leaky gut" by breaking apart the tight junctions between gut cells. This allows partially digested food particles, microbes, and toxins to escape into the bloodstream, triggering inflammation.

- **Autoimmune Response**: The body recognizes these foreign particles as dangers once they enter the bloodstream and launches an autoimmune reaction to combat them. This may eventually progress to other autoimmune diseases like celiac disease.

- **Microbiome Disruption**: It has been demonstrated that gluten decreases helpful species like Bifidobacteria and Lactobacillus while increasing populations of pathogenic bacteria like Enterobacteriaceae. Innervation is fueled by this dysbiosis.

- **Nutrient Malabsorption**: Gluten can harm the microvilli lining the intestinal walls and reduce the body's ability to absorb important vitamins, minerals, and antioxidants, even in people who are not celiac.

Be sure to carefully read labels as many innocent-looking goods, such as soy sauce, dressings, and seasonings, may contain gluten. Steer clear of all sources for at least 30 days to promote optimal gut healing.

Dairy

Dairy products and cow's milk are also frequently irritating to sensitive stomachs because of two main causes:

Lactose: Most adults lose their capacity to effectively digest lactose, the natural sugar found in dairy products, as they age. Gas, bloating, cramps, and diarrhea are brought on by this. Casein is one of the proteins that can cause problems even with lactose-free goods.

Casein and Whey Proteins: For many people, these dairy proteins cause severe allergies and inflammation. The body experiences allergic and autoimmune reactions once they are released through intestinal permeability. Mucus production may also be increased by casein.

Furthermore, compared to its raw equivalents, modern pasteurized dairy has comparatively less of the advantageous bacteria and enzymes that promote intestinal health.

For a minimum of 30 days, avoid any dairy products made from cow's milk, such as cheese, yogurt, ice cream, and whey supplements, to optimize the healing of your stomach. Later on, you can gradually bring back unsweetened cultured dairy products like kefir and yogurt as well as ghee, which is clarified butter that has had the milk particles removed.

Sugar

We all know that too much sugar wreaks havoc on our waistlines and blood sugar levels. But did you know added sugars also directly disrupt our gut microbiome? Here's how:

Prebiotic Effect: Refined sugars act as prebiotics that feed and promote the growth of harmful yeasts and opportunistic bacteria like Candida and E.coli. This crowds out the beneficial microbes.

Bacterial Overgrowth: Excessive sugar leads to bacterial overgrowth in the small intestine, generating high levels of toxic byproducts like methane gas. This can damage gut tissues.

Immune Disruption: Sugar suppresses immune function and antimicrobial defenses in the gut lining, allowing pathogens to thrive and cause periodic infections and diarrhea.

Pro-Inflammatory: Sugar triggers the release of inflammatory messengers called cytokines, contributing to leaky gut and inflammation throughout the body.

You'll want to steer clear of not just obvious sugar sources like candy, soda, and desserts, but also hidden sugars lurking in condiments, dressings, and processed foods. Always scrutinize labels for any syrups, cane sugar, dextrose, sucrose, etc.

Other Common Gut Irritants

Here are some additional food items to limit or avoid on a gut healing protocol:

Processed Foods: Loaded with inflammatory vegetable oils, additives, artificial sweeteners, and refined flours, these lack nutritional value yet incite gut dysfunction.

Soy Products: Many individuals develop sensitivities to proteins found in non-fermented soy foods like soy milk, veggie burgers, and protein powders.

Conventional Meats and Eggs: Choose grass-fed, pastured varieties to avoid antibiotics, hormones, and toxins that harm gut flora.

Alcohol and Caffeine: Both are gut irritants that trigger inflammation, disrupt nutrient absorption and exacerbate leaky gut.

Fried Foods and Vegetable Oils: Hydrogenated oils like corn, soybean, and sunflower oils promote oxidative stress and inflammation.

Pay attention to your body's needs and be aware of any dietary sensitivity or intolerances you may have to any of the items listed above. You can find out what your gut triggers are and how to avoid them by following an elimination diet for two to four weeks.

Recall that this is a temporary removal meant to reduce inflammation and reset your digestive system, not a life sentence. You can probably reintroduce modest amounts of such meals as tolerated with time and healing. But be ready to find new favorite foods and routines and make long-lasting lifestyle changes.

It takes self-awareness, perseverance, and making supportive internal environments through food choices to have a happy, healthy gut. Think of this as the beginning of a lifetime path to bright wellness!

Focusing on Anti-Inflammatory Foods, Fiber, Fermented Foods

The majority of digestive disorders and a host of other health conditions are caused by chronic inflammation. You may create an ideal environment for gut healing by include enough of anti-inflammatory meals, enough fiber, and healthful fermented foods.

Anti-Inflammatory Foods

There are foods that can seal a damaged, leaky gut lining and reduce inflammation. Make an effort to incorporate as many of these meals as you can:

Fruits and Vegetables: Eat an abundance of colorful produce, such as tomatoes, pumpkins, carrots, leafy greens, berries, and cherries. The wide range of antioxidants (carotenoids, anthocyanins, vitamin C, etc.) lessens oxidative stress and neutralizes free radicals.

Omega-3s These healthy fats are found in oily fish, walnuts, chia, and flax, and their oils dampen inflammation. They also enhance gut barrier function and benefit the gut microbiome.

Spices and Herbs Many common spices are potent anti-inflammatories. Ginger, turmeric, cumin, rosemary, garlic, thyme, oregano, and cayenne suppress inflammatory compounds like cytokines and prostaglandins.

Green Tea Due to the EGCG compound, green tea delivers powerful antioxidant and anti-inflammatory effects. It protects against leaky gut and oxidative stress.

Bone Broth Simmering animal bones into a nutrient-rich broth provides gut-healing proteins like collagen, gelatin, glycine, and glutamine. These nutrients seal holes and repair intestinal lining damage.

Anti-Inflammatory Supplements Supplements like fish oil, curcumin (turmeric), spirulina, ginger, grape seed extract, and resveratrol offer targeted anti-inflammatory benefits for the gut.

High Fiber Foods

Dietary fiber is crucial fuel for the beneficial gut bacteria. Insufficient fiber leads to gut dysbiosis and inflammation. The microbes ferment fiber to produce anti-inflammatory short-chain fatty acids that nourish gut cells.

Aim for 25-30 grams of dietary fiber per day from varied sources like:

- Vegetables (artichoke, broccoli, Brussels sprouts, carrots)
- Fruits (avocado, berries, pears, oranges)

- Legumes (lentils, beans, edamame)
- Nuts and seeds (flax, chia, almonds, pistachios)
- Whole grains (oats, brown rice, quinoa)
- Sources of inulin fiber (onions, garlic, leeks)

Increase fiber intake slowly to allow the gut to adapt. Stay well hydrated and physically active to facilitate smooth digestion.

Fermented Foods

These time-honored foods provide a concentrated source of probiotics - live bacteria beneficial for gut health. Including a variety in your diet can help replenish the gut with diverse microbial populations.

Yogurt and Kefir Look for varieties made with live active cultures, minimal sugar, and grass-fed dairy milk or non-dairy milk like coconut or almond. Greek and Skyr yogurt tend to be higher in protein.

Sauerkraut and Kimchi Made by fermenting cabbage and other veggies, these traditional foods are rich in lactobacillus strains that boost digestion and immunity. Look for unpasteurized versions.

Kombucha This fizzy fermented tea contains a colony of different yeasts and bacteria that aid digestion and liver function. Try fruit-flavored varieties for more taste.

Other fermented foods Miso, tempeh, natto, pickles, fermented vegetables, kvass, apple cider vinegar, sourdough bread, and aged cheeses are also rich in probiotics.

Start slowly with fermented foods, like a tablespoon per day, and gradually increase portions. This allows your gut to adapt to the influx of new bacterial species.

Probiotic Supplements
While supplements cannot fully replicate the diversity of food sources, they provide a concentrated probiotic boost. The best options contain 30-100 billion CFU and multiple strains like:

- Lactobacillus (acidophilus, rhamnosus, plantarum)
- Bifidobacterium (bifidum, longum, breve)
- Saccharomyces (boulardii yeast)

It's advisable to rotate different probiotic products regularly to support gut microbial diversity. Always pair probiotics with adequate fiber or prebiotic foods which provide their fuel source.

Prebiotics These specialized plant fibers serve as fertilizer for probiotics. The top prebiotic sources are onions, garlic, asparagus, bananas, apples, cocoa, flaxseeds, and chicory root. Jerusalem artichokes and yacón syrup are especially rich in prebiotics.

By focusing your diet on anti-inflammatory foods, plentiful fiber, fermented items, and pre/probiotics, you create an intestinal environment ripe for the proliferation of beneficial gut flora. This helps resolve inflammation, seal intestinal permeability, and restore optimal digestion.

Sample Meal Plan and Recipes

Adopting a gut-friendly diet can seem daunting at first, but with a little planning and creativity, it becomes a delicious and sustainable lifestyle. Here is a 7-day meal plan with recipes to get you started on reclaiming your gut health.

Week 1 Meal Plan

Day 1

- Breakfast: Coconut kefir smoothie with spinach, mango and chia seeds
- Lunch: Massaged kale salad with garbanzo beans, avocado, olive oil lemon dressing
- Dinner: Baked wild salmon with roasted Brussels sprouts and sweet potato wedges

Day 2

- Breakfast: Greek yogurt with mixed berries, sliced almonds, and a drizzle of honey
- Lunch: Hearty vegetable soup (recipe below) with a side salad
- Dinner: Grilled chicken kabobs with bell peppers, zucchini, red onion

Day 3

- Breakfast: Oven-baked sweet potato hash with spinach, eggs and avocado
- Lunch: Tuna stuffed avocado boats over mixed greens

- Dinner: Slow cooker bone broth chicken vegetable soup (recipe below)

Day 4

- Breakfast: Veggie frittata muffins with roasted tomatoes
- Lunch: Quinoa tabbouleh salad with chickpeas and lemon vinaigrette
- Dinner: Baked cod with mashed cauliflower and sautéed garlicky greens

Day 5

- Breakfast: Overnight chia seed pudding with coconut milk and berries
- Lunch: Lettuce wraps with sliced turkey breast, avocado and tomato
- Dinner: Zucchini noodles with pesto shrimp and roasted beets

Day 6

- Breakfast: Smoothie bowl with blended avocado, kale and almond milk
- Lunch: Leftover bone broth veggie soup from day 3
- Dinner: Grilled bison burgers lettuce wrapped with sauerkraut and sweet potato fries

Day 7

- Breakfast: Baked avocado boats with salsa and eggs

- Lunch: Loaded sweet potato with black beans, salsa, guacamole
- Dinner: Spaghetti squash with turkey meat sauce and a side salad

As you can see, the meals emphasize prebiotic-rich vegetables, healthy proteins, fermented foods, and soothing beverages to nourish your gut. Let's look at a few delicious recipes:

1. Hearty Vegetable Soup

Ingredients:

- 2 tbsp olive oil or ghee
- 1 onion, diced
- 3 carrots, sliced
- 3 stalks celery, sliced
- 1 cup mushrooms, sliced
- 6 cups vegetable or bone broth
- 1 can diced tomatoes
- 1 tsp dried oregano
- Salt and pepper to taste
- 2 cups greens like kale or spinach
- 1/4 cup parsley, chopped

Instructions:

1. In a large pot, heat oil/ghee over medium heat. Sauté onions for 2 minutes.
2. Add carrots, celery and mushrooms. Cook for 5 minutes, stirring frequently.
3. Pour in broth, tomatoes, oregano, and seasonings. Bring to a boil.
4. Reduce heat and simmer for 15 minutes.
5. Add greens and parsley, cooking for 2 more minutes.
6. Serve warm, optionally topped with avocado or sauerkraut.

2. Slow Cooker Bone Broth Veggie Soup

Ingredients:

- 1 whole pastured chicken or bones
- 8 cups water
- 2 tbsp apple cider vinegar
- 1 onion, quartered
- 3 carrots, halved
- 3 celery stalks, halved
- 2 inches fresh turmeric, peeled (or 1 tsp powder)
- 1 bunch parsley
- Salt and pepper to taste

Instructions:

1. Place all ingredients in the crockpot and cook on low for 18-24 hours.
2. Carefully remove chicken if using a whole bird.
3. Strain and discard bones/vegetables.
4. Shred chicken if desired and add the meat back to the broth.
5. Adjust seasoning as needed. Can add greens, zucchini, etc.

3. Gut-Healing Green Smoothie

Ingredients:

- 1 cup coconut milk or kefir
- 1 cup baby spinach
- 1/2 avocado
- 1/2 cup frozen mango or pineapple
- 1 tbsp chia seeds or ground flax
- 1-inch grated ginger (or 1/2 tsp powder)
- 1/4 cup parsley or cilantro
- 1 tsp spirulina powder (optional)
- Stevia or honey to sweeten if desired

Instructions:

1. Blend all ingredients until smooth.
2. Add water as needed to reach the desired consistency.

3. Top with bee pollen, coconut flakes, or cacao nibs.

4. Coconut Kefir Chia Pudding

Ingredients:

- 1 cup coconut milk kefir
- 1/4 cup chia seeds
- 1 tsp vanilla extract
- 1 tbsp honey (optional)
- 1/2 cup fresh berries
- 2 tbsp slivered almonds

Instructions:

1. In a jar or bowl, mix the kefir, chia seeds, vanilla, and honey (if using).
2. Cover and refrigerate for at least 4 hours or overnight to allow the chia to thicken.
3. Top with fresh berries and slivered almonds before serving.

5. Turmeric Bone Broth

Ingredients:

- 3 lbs beef or chicken bones
- 1 onion, quartered
- 2 carrots, cut into chunks
- 2 celery stalks, cut into chunks

- 1-inch knob fresh turmeric, sliced
- 1 tbsp apple cider vinegar
- 1 tsp whole peppercorns
- Filtered water to cover
- Sea salt to taste

Instructions:

1. Place all ingredients in a large pot and cover with filtered water by 1-2 inches.
2. Bring to a boil, then reduce heat and simmer for 12-24 hours, skimming foam occasionally.
3. Strain and discard bones/veggies.
4. Allow broth to cool slightly and pour into jars or containers. Refrigerate for up to 5 days.

6. Beet and Goat Cheese Arugula Salad

Ingredients:

- 4 cups arugula
- 4 medium beets, roasted and diced
- 1/2 cup crumbled goat cheese
- 1/4 cup pumpkin seeds
- 2 tbsp olive oil
- 1 tbsp balsamic vinegar
- Sea salt and pepper to taste

Instructions:

1. In a bowl, toss together arugula, roasted beets, goat cheese, and pumpkin seeds.
2. Drizzle with olive oil and balsamic vinegar.
3. Season with salt and pepper to taste.

7. Cauliflower Rice Tabbouleh

Ingredients:

- 1 head cauliflower, riced
- 1 cup parsley, chopped
- 1/2 cup mint leaves, chopped
- 1/4 cup olive oil
- 2 tbsp lemon juice
- 1 cup cherry tomatoes, halved
- 1/2 red onion, diced
- Sea salt and pepper to taste

Instructions:

1. Place riced cauliflower in a bowl with chopped parsley and mint.
2. In a small bowl, whisk together olive oil, lemon juice, salt, and pepper.
3. Pour dressing over cauliflower and toss to coat.
4. Gently fold in cherry tomatoes and red onion.

8. Zucchini Noodles with Avocado Sauce

Ingredients:

- 4 zucchinis, spiralized into noodles
- 2 avocados
- 1/4 cup fresh basil
- 2 cloves garlic
- 2 tbsp lemon juice
- 1/4 cup olive oil
- 1/4 cup water or broth
- Sea salt and pepper to taste
- Cherry tomatoes and pine nuts for topping

Instructions:

1. Make the avocado sauce by blending avocados, basil, garlic, lemon, olive oil, water, and salt/pepper until smooth.
2. In a skillet, sauté zucchini noodles for 2-3 minutes until just tender.
3. Toss noodles with avocado sauce and top with cherry tomatoes and pine nuts.

9. Anti-inflammatory Turmeric Smoothie

Ingredients:

- 1 frozen banana

- 1 cup unsweetened almond milk
- 1 tbsp almond butter
- 1 tsp ground turmeric
- 1/2 tsp ground ginger
- 1/4 tsp cinnamon
- 1 tbsp honey or maple syrup
- Ice cubes as needed

Instructions:

1. Add all ingredients to a blender and blend until completely smooth.
2. Add more almond milk to reach the desired consistency.
3. Pour into a glass and enjoy!

10. Kale Chips

Ingredients:

- 1 large bunch kale, washed and dried
- 2 tbsp olive oil or avocado oil
- 1/2 tsp sea salt
- 1 tsp nutritional yeast (optional)

Instructions:

1. Preheat oven to 275°F. Line baking sheets with parchment paper.

2. Remove kale leaves from stems and tear them into large pieces. Toss with oil, salt, and nutritional yeast if using.

3. Spread kale in a single layer across baking sheets.

4. Bake for 18-22 minutes, rotating pans halfway through until kale is crispy.

These nutrient-dense recipes provide plenty of fiber, healthy fats, antioxidants, and probiotics to nourish your microbiome. Be creative with herbs, spices, and different vegetable combinations!

The key is to eat as many whole, unprocessed foods as possible that are rich in fiber, nutrients, anti-inflammatories, and probiotics. Get creative with spices, fresh herbs, and simple preparations. Listen to your body and adjust ingredients as needed. With time and consistency, your gut health will flourish on this nourishing diet!

Conclusion

As we conclude this chapter on a nourishing gut health diet, it's crucial to reiterate the importance of making this a sustainable lifestyle change. Diets don't work in the long run - only a shift in your overall eating habits and relationship with food will create a lasting transformation.

Building on the knowledge you've gained, here are some key takeaways and strategies to seamlessly transition to a gut-friendly way of eating:

Be Prepared

One major pitfall when changing dietary habits is a lack of preparation. Take time to declutter your pantry and refrigerator of inflammatory trigger foods like gluten, dairy, sugar, processed snacks, and vegetable oils. Restock with an abundance of fresh produce, proteins, gut-healing ingredients like bone broth, and probiotic foods.

Invest in meal prep containers and cook batches of easy grab-and-go items like:

- Hard-boiled eggs
- Pre-cooked proteins (chicken, salmon)
- Chopped veggies
- Single-portion nut/seed mixes
- Gut-healing smoothies and drinks

Having nourishing options readily available prevents you from resorting to fast food or unhealthy choices when hunger strikes.

Start Slow

Ease into your new diet instead of drastically overhauling your entire eating regimen overnight. This can feel restrictive and lead to burnout. Begin with simple swaps like:

- Choose zucchini noodles over wheat pasta
- Use lettuce wraps instead of sandwich bread
- Swap cow's milk for unsweetened almond or coconut milk
- Snack on nuts and seeds instead of chips
- Cook with coconut oil or ghee over vegetable oils

Every small change makes a difference in reducing inflammation and nurturing your microbiome.

Explore New Recipes and Flavors

This dietary approach opens up a world of exciting new recipes, flavors, and ingredients to experiment with, preventing taste boredom. Look for new recipes using:

- Ancient grains (quinoa, amaranth, millet)
- Gut-friendly flours (almond, coconut, cassava)
- Different fermented foods (kimchi, miso, kefir)
- Flavorful spice blends (Cajun, Indian masalas)
- Fresh herbs (cilantro, parsley, basil, dill)
- Interesting produce (jicama, kohlrabi, rutabaga)
- Alternative protein sources (bison, lamb, tempeh)

Peruse ethnic grocery stores and farmers' markets for novel items to infuse variety into your meals. Don't forget to treat yourself to special gut-healing treats like coconut milk gelato occasionally as well!

Get Your Family Involved

Switching to a gut-friendly lifestyle becomes so much easier when your loved ones are on board and supportive. Gradually introduce new recipes and foods to your family and solicit their feedback and preferences. Let them pick out new items at the grocery store and get hands-on with cooking.

Making mealtimes an enjoyable bonding experience prevents the feelings of deprivation that often derail new dietary changes. With consistency, your family's tastebuds will adapt, and gut-healing foods will become second nature.

Prioritize Self-Care

Healing your gut requires nurturing both the body and the mind. Be sure to incorporate stress management techniques like breathwork, journaling, spending time in nature, and getting quality sleep. Chronic stress directly impairs the gut-brain connection and keeps inflammation firing.

Additionally, make movement and physical activity a non-negotiable part of your routine for optimal digestion, motility, and microbiome health.

Be Patient and Persevere

It's important to have realistic expectations as you undertake this profound dietary shift. Everybody is different in their healing timeline and response. While some experience dramatic relief within days of changing their diet, others require more sustained effort.

However, you can trust that if you adhere to the principles of gut-healthy eating covered in this chapter, your microbiome will eventually re-balance. Stay consistent, listen to your body's signals, and make tweaks as needed. Healing is a journey, but an incredibly rewarding one!

You now have a comprehensive roadmap to feed your gut the nutrients, probiotics, fiber, and healing foods it craves while eliminating inflammatory triggers. With dedication, you CAN overcome chronic gut issues, strengthen digestion, resolve nagging symptoms, and reclaim your vitality.

Your gut microbes influence countless aspects of your health - they impact everything from immunity and hormones to mental clarity and emotional balance. By nurturing this pivotal community within you, you pave the way for a lifetime of well-being from the inside out. Stay the course, and be amazed at the positive shifts!

Chapter 5: Lifestyle Changes for Better Gut Health

Now that we've laid the groundwork for empowering digestive health and balanced hormones through purposeful nutrition, it's time to explore complimentary lifestyle shifts and routines carrying these efforts to their fullest potential.

Within this chapter, we delve into practical and sustainable wellness practices shown through research to support gut resilience from both physical and emotional vantage points. Small everyday choices compound tremendously over time to nourish your inner world in a relaxing yet rejuvenating manner.

You'll discover natural stress management strategies, optimal sleep hygiene, exercises tailored to your needs, and tools for riding out life's ebbs and flows with grace. Combined with a nourishing plant-focused diet, these lifestyle considerations gift profoundly empowering well-being from the inside out while aging beautifully.

With insight and care for your continuously evolving radiance, allow these recommendations to inspire as you determine personalized adjustments aligning mind, body, and spirit. Your pathway awaits - may this chapter light the way toward sustained balance, harmony, and health through everyday self-nurturance. Onwards to vibrant living!

Managing stress and cortisol levels

With aging comes an accumulation of daily demands placing wear on mind and body alike. Yet stress management proves so vital for balanced gut function and hormones at this life stage. Here are evidence-backed approaches:

- Mild exercises and meditation cultivate mindfulness lowering physiological stress responses. Commit to just 10 minutes daily.

- Spend time in nature through gardening, hiking or simply gazing at trees. Interacting with nature reduces cortisol while boosting mood.

- Practice relaxing compassionate self-talk and challenge negative thoughts triggering the stress response unnecessarily.

- Prioritize downtime through soothing baths, reading, crafts, and socializing with loved ones providing emotional fulfillment.

- Employ coping tools like essential oil blends, calming teas, therapeutic breathing, and gratitude journaling to soothe tension daily.

- Express emotions healthily through creative outlets like art, music, journaling, or calling a trusted friend rather than internalizing pressures.

- Establish boundaries to avoid taking on more than reasonably manageable energy levels and capacity. It's OK to say no.

By weaving these lifestyle habits addressing mind, body, and spirit into your routine, you diffuse cortisol's long-term damaging influence naturally from within through peace of mind.

Getting regular exercise and restorative sleep

Quality movement coupled with sufficient rest forms the backbone of inner homeostasis and health span. Prioritize these self-care pillars with these action steps:

- Aim for 30 minutes daily of any activity enjoyed like walking, water aerobics, or home workouts. Gentle exertion aids digestion, mood, and immunity.

- Practice relaxation techniques before bed like reading, stretching, or Journaling to unwind mentally. Limit screen time for natural melatonin secretion.

- Establish a calming, dark, and comfortable sleep space free of stress-inducing stimuli supporting strong circadian rhythms.

- Stick to a consistent schedule by going to bed and waking up within the same 1-2 hour window daily, even on weekends.

- Address any sleep disruptors like pain, noise, or caffeine through targeted solutions to optimize 7-9 hours nightly for balanced hormones.

- If needing restorative catch-up, Schedule short naps or slow Sunday mornings under one hour to avoid daytime grogginess.

- Consume evening meals light in protein and carbs while staying hydrated to avoid indigestion interrupting sleep.

Nourishing your body with quality movement and rest lays the groundwork for vibrant energy levels, digestion, and resilience within your unique rhythm.

Supporting gut microbes through meditation, nature

While diet and stress relief impact gut flora profoundly, lifestyle habits can directly interact with microbial populations as well. Two nourishing practices in particular provide bottom-up renewal:

Mindful meditation

Just 10 minutes daily of focused breathwork and presence lowers cortisol stressing symbionts. Research shows meditation may reinforce biodiversity by calming the mind-gut axis.

Beginning meditators can start simply by focusing on natural breaths and gently redirecting wandering thoughts. Apps provide basic guided sessions too. Consistency breeds benefits compounding over the lifespan.

Nature immersion

Spending structured time amid trees, plants, and natural environments encourages flourishing gut flora populations according to studies. The hypothesized mechanisms could involve:

- Reduced anxiety lifting stressors like cortisol disrupting microbe equilibrium.

- Exposure to diverse environmental microorganisms through light activities like gardening potentially populates our own GI tracts.

- Antimicrobial plant compounds and fibers contact intestinal cells signaling a relaxing, nourishing environment conducive to diversity.

Aim to gently move your body outdoors at a minimum once daily, even if just a brief walk with conscious awareness of your natural surroundings restoring wholeness. Each interaction supports inner balance and well-being.

Probiotics and prebiotics

While food sources provide the backbone for flourishing gut flora during this transition, targeted supplementation offers valuable support when life circumstances disrupt natural intake. Some suggestions:

- Pair a high-potency probiotic containing 30-50 billion live cultures taken refrigerated with a prebiotic fiber to fuel thriving microbes.

- Rotate supplement types housing different bacterial strains to reinforce diversity month to month. Common options include Lactobacillus, Bifidobacterium, and Saccharomyces boulardii.

- Schedule probiotic dosing with or after meals to facilitate contact with digestive juices and ensure colonies reach the lower intestines to colonize.

- Check expiration dates and storage, as heat and light degrade live bacteria quickly without proper refrigeration.

- For occasional digestive disruption, consider a Saccharomyces boulardii supplement shown to effectively reduce bloating, constipation, or diarrhea when cycling as needed alongside lifestyle adjustments.

Supplements judiciously support your inner garden during unavoidable stressors to help your gorgeous self flourish even through life's ebbs and flows. Combined with stress relief and nourishing foods, balanced bliss naturally follows.

Conclusion

And so here we are at the culmination of our journey exploring the profound capacity for radiant health and inner renewal through gentle yet focused gut-centered lifestyle medicine. I hope the insights, recommendations, and recipes shared have sparked inspiration and practical steps for nurturing your glowing well-being during this rich season of life.

While targeted nutrition, stress relief, and other daily empowerment tools form an integral foundation, I wish to reiterate that sustainable lifelong change emerges freely from within through compassion. May you embrace your beautiful humanity exactly as it uniquely unfolds moment to moment - through patience, curiosity, and grace both for yourself and all beings along parallel paths.

Your guts are but one aspect comprising the glorious whole that is you. May the connections drawn within these chapters serve to remind us of innate inner wisdom, resilience, and the ability to expertly craft each day according to your highest good. Go forth in radiance, courage, and care for your divine self!

Key takeaways

As we reflect on lessons gleaned to carry into your next chapter of vibrant gut-nourishing self-care, let's summarize a few vital pieces of wisdom:

- Your diet forms the foundation dictating digestive health and hormonal harmony. Focus on high-fiber whole foods rich in antioxidants.

- Gentle yet consistent lifestyle practices like movement, restorative sleep, meditation and social interaction safeguard resilience amidst change.

- Managing daily stressors through compassionate mindfulness, grounding activities, and expressing emotions enrich well-being on deep levels over the years.

- Honoring your intuition by listening to your body's subtle cues, keeping a food journal, and adjusting patterns accordingly supports vibrant longevity.

- Surrounding yourself with uplifting people, hobbies, and environments nurtures mental health hand in hand with physical care.

- Having patience, self-kindness and maintaining gratitude for each step shaped this journey into transformational self-empowerment and radiance from within.

- Your growth continues freely as an exciting lifelong discovery. May your inner light shine ever brighter!

Wishing you much health, joy and empowerment as your gut-centered revolution unfolds. Remember that you've got this with compassionate consistency. Go in peace, beauty, and balance.

Putting it all together for an optimal gut reset

Now that we've covered fundamental lifestyle shifts supporting gut health at this empowering phase, let's synthesize key steps for a comprehensive reset plan tailored uniquely for you:

- Gradually implement the whole foods-based anti-inflammatory diet with prebiotics, probiotics, and bone broth daily over 4 weeks.

- Commit to 30 minutes of movement, 8 hours of sleep, and twice-daily meditations or relaxation techniques for balanced stress buffers.

- Gradually eliminate dietary triggers through journaling as discussed for 4 weeks before slowly reintroducing to discern sensitivities.

- Incorporate weekly fermented foods and limit processed foods for resilient microbes.

- Practice self-compassion through daily self-care rituals like baths, creative expression, and quality social time.

- Supplement intelligently with a broad-spectrum probiotic, prebiotic, and digestive enzymes as needed.

- Re-evaluate your routine regularly, adapting new insights for continuous evolution customized to your experience.

- Celebrate non-scale victories like stable moods and sustainable energy levels emerging through patience.

By steadfastly yet gently aligning your unique environment, diet, and lifestyle, long-term gut and whole-body balance radiantly follows. Wishing you much empowerment on your journey ahead!

Looking ahead to healthier aging

As you've gained insights into cultivating balanced gut function and hormonal harmony presently, maintaining focus inward grants even deeper rewards as the years unfold. Some forward-looking reflections:

- Prioritizing nourishing self-care preserves wellness capital to face inevitable future challenges with grace and resilience.

- Continued gut diversity supports strong immunity against infections as exposure increases within the community.

- Gut-nourishing lifestyle habits and stress resilience counter the impacts of cellular aging at a deep, protective level over decades.

- Daily mindfulness keeps stress hormones in healthy check to avoid inflammation heightening age-related illness risk.

- Nourishing nutrition packed with antioxidants wards off oxidative damage acutely worsening with time if left unchecked.

- Physical activity, social engagement and purposeful living stave off decline by maintaining connections in body and mind.

While aging brings change, your capacity to thrive endures through ongoing compassionate empowerment from within. May your radiance only deepen with wisdom and experience. Wishing you a vibrant journey ahead in the health of body and spirit!

About the Author

A passionate advocate for holistic health and wellness, Dr. Omolola Habib leverages her background in Naturopathic Medicine and extensive experience as a wellness coach to dedicate her career to guiding individuals to achieve optimal health through natural means.

The intersection of gut health and hormonal balance, particularly in women over 50, represents Dr. Habib's area of expertise. With her profound understanding of the body's interconnected systems; she can offer practical--even effective--strategies for healing the gut and restoring hormonal equilibrium.

Dr. Habib, propelled by an authentic aspiration to enhance others' lives: she has indeed made a positive impact on numerous individuals. Her personalized approach to wellness manifests her commitment--a fervent dedication towards empowering others--in both her writing and guidance; thus reflecting not only professional excellence but also a heartfelt desire for people taking control of their health.

Dr. Habib, the author of "Gut Reset for Women: A Holistic Guide to Heal Your Stomach and Balance Hormones After 50," actively shares her wealth of knowledge and insights; she intends this book not merely as a source of information but as an inspiration for readers--a catalyst propelling them towards vibrant health and well-being. Specifically targeting women, she endeavors through these pages to foster understanding: it is time we all start embracing natural solutions—be they dietary changes or lifestyle adjustments—for digestive issues, hormonal imbalances, and overarching wellness; because at its core lays our body's innate ability to heal itself when given proper care & attention.

A trusted resource for those seeking to transform their health and reclaim vitality at any age, Dr. Omolola Habib combines her expertise in Naturopathic Medicine with a compassionate approach.

www.ingramcontent.com/pod-product-compliance
Lightning Source LLC
Chambersburg PA
CBHW070408230526
45471CB00006B/2706